Natural Alternatives

TO HRT

Overcome Osteoporosis, Heart Disease
and Other Menopausal Conditions
without Risky Synthetic
Hormone Replacement

RITA ELKINS, M.H.

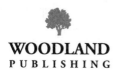

WOODLAND
PUBLISHING

For ordering or other information, please contact us:
Woodland Publishing
448 East 800 North
Orem, Utah 84097
Visit us at our web site: www.woodlandpublishing.com
or call us toll-free: (800) 777-2665

The information in this book is for educational purposes only and is not recommended as a means of diagnosing or treating an illness. All matters regarding physical and mental health should be supervised by a health practitioner knowledgeable in treating that particular condition. Neither the publisher nor the author directly or indirectly dispenses medical advice, nor do they prescribe any remedies or assume any responsibility for those who choose to treat themselves.

ISBN 1-58054-369-3
Printed in the United States of America

Contents

Introduction: The End of the Estrogen Era

In mid-July 2002, news services dropped a medical bombshell. After five years of research, scientists in charge of one of the largest federally funded studies on hormone replacement therapy (HRT) concluded that the risks of HRT outweighed its benefits. The study, which was part of a larger fifteen-year trial by the National Heart, Lung and Blood Institute called the Women's Health Initiative (WHI), was cut short because the data clearly showed that women taking HRT therapy (such as Prempro) had a greater risk (over 25 percent higher) of developing breast cancer. Moreover, heart attack risk increased 29 percent, stroke by 41 percent and blood clot rates were doubled compared with those who did not take these drugs.

Due to mounting concern, the study—which was originally slated to last over eight years and involved over sixteen thousand women—was abruptly halted after only five years. Ironically, this study looked at the safety of estrogen/progestin combination drugs, which were supposed to be infinitely safer than taking estrogen alone. This perception proved to be wrong. Yet last year alone, American pharmacists filled over forty million prescriptions for Premarin and over twenty million for Prempro (the same drug with added progestins).

So what happens now? Should all women go off of hormone therapy even for short-term problems like hot flashes? If you do stop HRT, are there any natural compounds that effectively protect the heart and bones of postmenopausal women? And what about young women who have had hysterectomies? Should they continue with their HRT programs? If you are one of the more than six million women in this country who take an estrogen and progestin combination (like Prempro) for a variety of reasons, this booklet is for you.

The Perils of HRT

Before a woman can decide what is best for her hormonal future, she needs to acquaint herself with some little-known facts that she probably won't hear from her doctor. Fiddling around with HRT is serious business and should not be taken lightly. The casual use of HRT in its various forms can pose serious health risks. First, let's look at the reasons that doctors sometimes advise HRT use (or have advised it in the past).

REASONS WOMEN TAKE HRT

1. To protect them from heart disease.

Just the opposite appears to be the case.

2. To stabilize mood and emotions.

Depression and irritability can occur with HRT therapy.

3. To keep bones strong and prevent osteoporosis.

Although HRT may offer some protection, it does not create new bone stores and may even promote bone loss.

4. To preserve memory and keep mental function sharp.

New studies contradict this effect. Estrogen does not decrease your risk of Alzheimer's disease.

5. To treat hot flashes, vaginal dryness and other menopausal symptoms.

There are other ways to accomplish this with little or no health risks.

HORMONE REPLACEMENT RISKS

HRT also carries significant risks, which may outweigh its benefits. It may increase your risk of

- breast cancer
- gallbladder disease
- blood clots
- heart attack and stroke

HRT has also been associated with

- liver dysfunction
- breast tenderness
- increased risk of birth defects
- acne

- insomnia
- increased fat storage
- headaches
- decreased sex drive
- bone loss

- swelling and fluid retention
- depression
- impaired blood sugar control
- fibroids

Conclusion: HRT therapy does more damage than good. (Alternative care practitioners have been saying this for years.)

HRT AND HEART DISEASE: SEPARATING FACT FROM FICTION

Does estrogen raise good cholesterol, thereby reducing your risk of postmenopausal heart disease? Recent studies from both the National Institutes of Health (NIH) and the *Journal of the American Medical Association* (*JAMA*) on estrogen/progestin combo drugs have failed to support this once-believed notion. In fact, just the opposite may actually be the case—talk about irony. New trials have shown that when a woman takes HRT for more than about five years, her risk of heart disease actually increases.

As a result, the American Heart Association's president, Robert Bonow, M.D., said in a recently released press advisory, "Based on current evidence, the American Heart Association (AHA) advises that women do not start or continue combined HRT for the prevention of coronary artery disease" (July 9, 2002). This advisory expands the 2001 update warning postmenopausal women with heart disease about HRT to include all postmenopausal women. Instead it advises that women focus on reducing their heart disease risk by controlling cholesterol and blood pressure through safer methods: a healthy diet, regular exercise and, if necessary, drug therapy. The AHA also maintains that if a woman chooses to use HRT for reasons other than heart health, she should use it for the shortest time possible.

THE BREAST CANCER RISK

The million-dollar question—*does HRT cause more breast cancer?*—was addressed by the famous WHI study of more than sixteen thousand women. Not only does this study say HRT causes breast cancer, but another trial conducted in Sweden found that women taking estrogen therapy may quadruple their risk of developing breast cancer. In other words, women who took a combination of estrogen and progestin for more than six years were 4.4 times more likely to develop breast cancer.

Once again, the addition of progestin to help prevent breast cancer appears to have backfired. In fact, the combination of estrogen and progestin shows the highest risk of breast cancer. Another study published in a 1994 issue of *Molecular and Cellular Endocrinology* reported that synthetic progestins stimulate the proliferation of breast tumor cells.

HRT and Blood Clots

Long before the study of sixteen thousand women concluded that blood clots were a real concern, an earlier study called the Heart and Estrogen-Progestin Replacement Study (HERS), published in *JAMA*, concluded that women taking hormone therapy were up to three times more likely to develop blood clots than those taking a placebo.

HRT and Gallbladder Disease

Once again, the association of hormone therapy with an increased risk of gallbladder disease was also confirmed by recent findings. Although earlier studies suggested that women taking HRT were more likely to undergo gallbladder surgery, most of us would never think that taking synthetic hormones could negatively impact the gallbladder. What these findings suggest is that when hormonal drugs course through the bloodstream, every body system is affected.

HRT and Mood Control

Although many women take HRT for its supposed mood-enhancing effects, studies tell us that older women who took an estrogen/progestin drug did not experience an improvement in mood or emotional state. In fact, some women actually felt more irritable and depressed on HRT. Yet many women think that taking HRT is the only way to fight menopausal blues or mood swings. There are, however, several other much safer options to raise mood or control irritability that will be discussed later.

A CRASH COURSE IN CURRENT HRT FORMS

HRT has a multitude of names depending on its hormonal make-up. ERT (estrogen replacement therapy) refers to drugs consisting of estrogen only, such as Raloxifene. The most widely used estrogenic drug is called conjugated estrogen (better known as Premarin). Premarin is produced from the urine of pregnant mares and includes various forms of estrogen. PERT (progestin/estrogen replacement therapy) refers to drugs using a combination of both hormones, including Prempro and Premphase. While Estrace is produced from wild yam extract, it is still artificially synthesized. In short, conjugated estrogen (e.g., Premarin), estradiol (e.g., Estrace and Estraderm) or ethinyl estradiol (e.g., Alesse) and a progestin (e.g., Provera) are commonly prescribed.

PREMARIN: PANDORA'S BOX?

Premarin hit the market in 1942 and became the most-prescribed drug in America from 1992 through 1999. Last year alone, its manufacturer (Wyeth) reported sales that topped more than $2 billion. Thirty-eight percent of U.S. women between the ages of fifty and seventy-four take hormones after menopause, according to a national survey published in 1999.

PROGESTIN DRUGS ARE DANGEROUS

All women need to know that progestins are potent drugs that come with significant risks and side effects. Moreover, they are not remotely related to natural progesterone compounds. Progestins are artificially synthesized in a laboratory setting and are not well tolerated by the human body. Although they were originally thought to be safer than estrogen drugs alone, new data says otherwise.

Check out a few of the potential side effects listed in the *Physician's Desk Reference* (PDR) for the widely used HRT drug Provera:

- increased risk of birth defects, such as heart and limb defects, if taken during the first four months of pregnancy
- sudden or partial loss of vision
- possible development of malignant mammary nodules
- phlebitis, pulmonary embolism and cerebral thrombosis

- fluid retention
- breakthrough bleeding
- depression
- decreased glucose tolerance
- breast tenderness
- rashes
- unknown consequences if passed into breast milk

ALL HRT DELIVERY SYSTEMS ARE NOT CREATED EQUAL

At this writing, approximately 15 to 20 percent of post-menopausal women currently use some form of estrogen replacement therapy (a statistic that will undoubtedly take a rapid plunge in light of recent events). If you choose to remain on HRT, you will want to take the smallest possible dose. Moreover, you need to know that all delivery systems are not the same. Some forms of HRT are taken every day, others on certain days of the month, and still others are delivered through the skin by patches. Some experts believe that patches and vaginal hormone creams are safer because they skip the digestive route and directly enter the bloodstream. Moreover, when you take them off, the dosage immediately stops. On the other hand, oral HRT drugs are not readily eliminated from your system—increasing the likelihood of side effects and risks. Injections have the same drawback.

PLAYING THE HYSTERECTOMY CARD

If you are young and have had a hysterectomy, tell your doctor that you want a hormonal drug formula in proportions that most closely resemble what your body would have produced. Specify that you want to use the lowest possible therapeutic dosage, and stay away from estrogen/progesterone combinations. In addition, learn to use plant estrogens like soy isoflavones and natural progesterone to augment your therapy. Christine Conrad, co-author of *Natural Woman Natural Menopause* published in 1997, states that soy isoflavones and other plant estrogens can be effective hormone replacement agents for women who have had hysterectomies. Using soy isoflavones and natural progesterone cream is highly recommended.

Natural Alternatives to HRT for Menopause

Okay. The reports are in and phones are ringing off the hook in doctor's offices. We now have a landmark study that advises women to forgo long-term HRT use. So now what? In typical fashion, the medical community offers women no substitution for HRT, so women are on their own. Be assured, however, that there are several natural options that can certainly improve your hormonal landscape without risking your life. It only stands to reason that natural compounds which mimic female hormones have none of the side effects associated with artificial chemical imposters. Alternative practitioners have known this for years.

REPLACING ESTROGEN AND PROGESTERONE NATURALLY

Ideally, postmenopausal women should be using diet, exercise, phytoestrogens and natural progesterone to safeguard their bones and heart. There is also a growing consensus that the notion of taking hormones indefinitely after menopause is certainly not what nature intended. One is compelled to ask why Mother Nature did not arrange for women to make estrogens and progesterone until they die of old age. The widespread and even cavalier dispersal of synthetic hormones to women is causing an unprecedented backlash and for good reason. Women want the facts and have the right to weigh the pros and cons of any therapy. Unfortunately, the very valuable role of natural compounds has been grossly neglected.

JAPANESE WOMEN AND MENOPAUSE

Japanese women sail through menopause. They seem unaware of the phenomenon of hot flashes and night sweats. One study showed that over 50 percent of American and Western European women reported menopausal symptoms, while in Japan the number was less than 10 percent. The makeup of the Japanese diet may hold the secret to their hormonal health. Japanese women eat from 2.5 to 3.5 ounces of tofu per day (30 to 50 grams of soy protein daily), as opposed to the 1 to 3 grams consumed by women in the U.S. In fact, the urinary excretion of isoflavones in Japanese women is one hundred to one thousand times higher than in American women.

THE SOY SOLUTION FOR MENOPAUSE

Three recent studies looked at the effects of soy on post-menopausal women using soy protein isolate supplements, soy bars with (40 milligrams of phytoestrogens) and soy grits. The studies, which reported significant improvements, included one conducted in Australia with fifty-eight postmenopausal women who reported a 40 percent reduction in hot flashes. These women were consuming 45 grams of soy flour per day over a twelve-week period. Another trial conducted at the Royal Hospital for Women in Australia consisted of nine women who consumed 160 milligrams of isoflavones for twelve weeks and experienced a significant decrease in their number of hot flashes (from 6.7 to 3.4 per day). Still another British study found that giving 80 milligrams of isoflavones to a group of women for two months resulted in a significant decrease in the number of hot flashes.

An Australian research team concluded that soy isoflavones are likely to be therapeutically beneficial for women with mild to moderate menopausal symptoms. Italian research involving 104 postmenopausal women reported a significant reduction of 45 percent (versus 30 percent for the placebo substance) in the number of hot flashes after twelve weeks among women consuming 60 grams of soy protein isolate daily (containing 76 milligrams of isoflavones).

Moreover, researchers at Bowman Gray School of Medicine and Tufts conducted an eighteen-week study that examined the effects of soy on forty-three women (aged forty-five to fifty-five). For six weeks, the women added 20 grams (under 1 ounce, approximately 2 teaspoons) of powdered soy protein to their daily breakfast. For another six weeks, they added the same amount of soy protein to their diets, but split the amount into two 10-gram doses. For a third six-week period, they added a look-alike powdered carbohydrate placebo. Women taking soy reported significantly less severe hot flashes and night sweats. In addition, total cholesterol levels dropped an average of ten percent without any of the side effects seen with conventional hormonal therapy.

Soy Protects Against Cancer and Heart Disease

Unlike HRT, soy offers beneficial hormonal effects while lowering your risk of potentially fatal diseases. Show me a drug that does that? Something as simple as consuming 40 to 50 milligrams of isoflavones daily may be enough to obtain this dual benefit.

Soy and Postmenopausal Heart Disease

Prior to the release of research about the heart-related risks of HRT, one of the major reasons for choosing HRT was the belief it would help prevent heart disease (the number-one killer of women). In the past, most physicians told their patients that without HRT, a woman's risk of heart disease escalates. Once again, soy isoflavones seem tailor-made for menopausal women because they target virtually all major health concerns related to menopause, including heart disease.

A Japanese study published in 1998 involving close to five thousand test subjects reported that substantial soy consumption strongly correlated with lower cholesterol levels. Moreover, in a 1997 issue of *Fertility and Sterility*, data from a clinical study found that soy isoflavones appear to boost vascular function and protect the heart, suggesting that soy supplements may be an alternative to HRT for women concerned about their risk of heart attack.

Dr. Sulistiyani of the Primate Research Center at Bogor Agricultural University in Indonesia believes that the main reasons estrogen replacement therapy is so effective in helping to reduce the risk of coronary heart disease in postmenopausal women are its antioxidant properties. However, we already know that HRT is associated with an increased risk of certain cancers and can cause a whole host of unwanted side effects. In addition, one of the latest studies on HRT claims that it actually increased the risk of heart disease during the first year of its use.

On the other hand, soy has excellent antioxidant properties. A recent study using female monkeys who had their ovaries removed to simulate postmenopausal women showed that genistein inhibited LDL oxidation by 48 percent. When used in combination with vitamin E, this effect was even greater. What this study suggests is that soy protein offers powerful heart-protective properties for everyone and may be especially desirable for postmenopausal women who could also use its other estrogenic benefits.

Heart Healthy Soy: Cholesterol Buster

In 1995, the *New England Journal of Medicine* published an analysis of soy and concluded that "the consumption of soy protein rather than animal protein significantly decreased serum concentrations of total cholesterol, LDL cholesterol [the bad kind], and triglycerides, without significantly affecting serum HDL cholesterol [the good kind] concentrations." The review included thirty-eight controlled clinical trials. The average intake of soy protein was 47 grams per day, equivalent to the amount in one half cup of soy flour, and the average decrease in total cholesterol was 9.3 percent. This drop in blood cholesterol levels may seem small, but it represents a 20 to 30 percent reduction in heart disease risk.

Keep in mind that when cholesterol is artificially lowered with drugs, often the good kind (HDL) as well as the bad kind (LDL) drops, which is not a good thing. In contrast, soy protein lowers only LDL cholesterol. In addition, soy appears to decrease the amount of cholesterol that is oxidized. Oxidized cholesterol can damage artery walls. One clinical trial found that people who ate soy every day for six months experienced a 50 percent reduction in oxidized blood cholesterol compared with those who didn't eat soy.

Postmenopausal Strokes and Soy

Wake Forest University researchers have found that soy phytoestrogens decreased the incidence of atherosclerosis in the carotid artery (something Premarin was thought to do). A blockage of this artery is a leading cause of stroke. Proponents of the study pointed out that stroke is the third leading cause of death for middle-aged and postmenopausal women. It was concluded that using soy phytoestrogens to prevent plaque deposits in the carotid artery may be the best way to lower stroke incidence in older women.

Are Soy Estrogens Strong Enough to Do the Job?

Many women have turned to HRT because they have been led to believe that anything natural is not potent enough to stimulate desirable effects in the body. Dr. Kenneth D. Setchell, an expert on soy isoflavones, points out that after soy isoflavones are consumed, they are digested by intestinal bacteria, absorbed from the intestinal tract and then metabolized in the liver. However, he points out that eating even relatively small amounts of soy protein can significantly raise levels of circulating phytoestrogens. Studies suggest that consistently eating certain forms of soy can maintain a steady state of phytoestrogens in the blood. Consuming 50 milligrams per day of total isoflavones resulted in what is assumed to be therapeutic levels of phytoestrogens, the most important of which is called genistein.

Protein Content of Soy Foods per Half-Cup Serving (from Highest to Lowest)

SOY FOOD	GRAMS OF SOY PROTEIN
soy protein concentrate (1 oz)	58.1
soy flour (defatted)	47.0
soy meal (defatted, raw)	45.0
soybeans (dry roasted)	39.6
tempeh	19.0
natto	17.7
soybeans (cooked)	16.6
tofu (raw, firm)	15.6
miso	11.8
tofu (raw, regular)	8.1
okara	3.2
soy milk	2.8

THE ISOFLAVONE CONTENT OF COMMON SOY FOODS

- One ounce of **soy chips or nuts** contains 42 milligrams of isoflavones.
- One hundred grams of **soy flour** contain 50 milligrams of isoflavones.
- Four ounces of **tofu** contain 80 milligrams of isoflavones.
- Eight ounces of **raw soy milk** contain 50 milligrams of isoflavones.
- Most **soy foods** contain 1 to 2 milligrams of the isoflavone genistein per gram.

Foods to incorporate into the diet include tofu, soy milk, soy chips, miso, soy flour, soy protein drinks, soy nuts and spreads. You can put soy powder into any or all baking recipes. Tofu can be whipped into dips, sauces, mashed potatoes, spreads, desserts, fillings, etc. (For more information, refer to recipe section.)

Soy protein concentrate can be an excellent source of isoflavones. Genistein is the primary isoflavone found in soy. The amount of genistein present averages from 0.48 to 1.51 milligrams per gram. Be aware that all soy protein products do not contain isoflavones. Some are actually removed through processing, so look for isoflavone content on the label, and if none is listed, call the manufacturer.

USING GENISTEIN IN SUPPLEMENT FORM

Doctors may tell you that there are no long-term studies on the effects of using genistein as an isolated supplement. Yet common sense dictates that if you're not going to eat soy foods, supplementation may be the only way to get this valuable isoflavone in your system. Genistein has been the subject of scores of clinical studies, and its benefits are supported by mountains of data.

Doctors like Duane Townsend, M.D., consider genistein to be one of the most exciting phytoestrogens available and don't hesitate to use it in supplement form. Dr. Townsend believes that Mother Nature provides women with both genistein and natural progesterone to safely and effectively protect hormone-sensitive tissue and treat hormone- driven symptoms in women of all ages. "I found this out after years of medical practice, and I'm like a squeaky wheel—getting out the word to my patients and colleagues who are smart enough to listen. I call genistein and progesterone the 'dynamic duo,' and in a time when so many women feel skittish about hormonal drugs, their day has come," says Dr. Townsend. He strongly advises all women to eat more soy foods, use appropriate supplements, and to waste no time in doing so. In his book, *A Maverick of Medicine Speaks to Women*, Dr. Townsend says:

> I like to refer to genistein as tofu in a pill. I believe taking it in supplement form is the next best thing to eating a diet rich in soy foods. I've found that genistein can work just as well as the Premarins and Estraces in terms of relieving the symptoms of PMS. I also use it in lieu of HRT (hormone replacement therapy) whenever a patient is willing. I believe that when combined with natural progesterone, genistein offers women a very appealing option. I don't hesitate to give genistein to my patients who are going through menopause or who have had hysterectomies or breast cancer. The data is compelling—overwhelmingly positive, and I'm in favor of it because it works and it's safe. Most soy foods contain about 1 to 2 mg of genistein per gram of protein. Supplemental genistein is an easy way to make sure you're getting the estrogen-blocking action you need on a daily basis. Many women will fail to consume the amount of soy they need to achieve good results and tissue protection.

Over two thousand clinical studies demonstrate that genistein acts as a desirable "weak" (less potent) estrogen in the body. It actually blocks the dangerous effects of more powerful estrogens by binding to receptor sites in the breast and other tissues—essentially stealing sites from potentially deadly estrogen. In other words, genistein mimics estrogen, and by doing so, acts as both an "anti-estrogen" (taking the place of dangerous estrogen in the body) and a phytoestrogen (providing extra estrogen for those with a deficit) on demand. Show me a drug with that kind of smarts!

Using Genistein for Hot Flashes and Vaginal Dryness and Itching

Recommended dosages of soy isoflavones are 35 milligrams of genistein plus 3 to 5 milligrams of daidzein (another soy isoflavone) daily. Most soy isoflavone products contain both isoflavones. Be aware that if you suffer from intense hot flashes or other symptoms, you may need to double the dosage or add natural progesterone to achieve desired results. Taking an acidophilus supplement helps to optimize isoflavone absorption. Taking quercitin and curcumin also potentiates the action of genistein. (Use an unscented vaginal lubricant for vaginal dryness and itching.)

Natural Remedies for Hot Flashes

In light of the negative findings reported in July 2002 on combo HRT drugs, many doctors have stressed that using a short-term course of the drugs—instead of the long-term course previously prescribed—to treat conditions like hot flashes poses little or no risks. Considering the track record of these medical practitioners, however, one has to wonder if HRT is ever safe, even if it is used for only a little while. The credibility of the medical community is now a major issue.

Wisdom dictates that using HRT for hot flashes should be the exception rather than the rule. Menopausal women need to realize that hot flashes are temporary, and while taking hormonal drugs may help to ease them, is it really the answer? A significant number of women with hot flashes fail to obtain relief by using HRT. One study revealed that not only did some women still have hot flashes, they actually fared worse than a comparison group of women who didn't take anything whatsoever. In fact, Asian women don't even have a word that refers to hot flashes. However, if you do feel that you need some drug therapy, ask you doctor to use a very low dose of estrogen (estradiol, 0.5 mg or less).

THE SOY SOLUTION

Most Japanese women eat three to four ounces of soy foods daily, which is about two servings of tofu, tempeh or soy milk. Soy protein contains isoflavones. Drinking 15 ounces of soy milk (about 2 cups) or 2 ounces of tofu daily may help to ease hot flashes. Scientists at the National Institute of Environmental Health Sciences found that postmenopausal women who ate several soy-based foods for sixty days had less hot flashes.

A NATURAL-REMEDY PROGRAM FOR HOT FLASHES

1. **Eat more soy or use soy isoflavone supplements.**
   Current studies suggest that soy products are a viable treatment for menopausal symptoms. Add soybeans, tofu, miso, soy milk and other soy products to your diet. (Red clover is also high in isoflavones and can be taken in supplement form. Refer to a later herbal section for more details.)

2. **Use a natural progesterone cream.**
   One double-blind trial found that using a topical natural progesterone cream resulted in a reduction in hot flashes in 83 percent of test subjects, compared with only 19 percent of those given a placebo.

3. **Don't smoke or drink.**
   Women who do either have more hot flashes. Cut back on coffee and other sources of caffeine. Caffeine can also worsen hot flashes.

4. **Use deep breathing exercises to control hot flashes.**
   A recent study revealed that women who engage in deep-breathing exercises were able to reduce their hot flashes by 50 percent.

5. **Wear cotton clothing.**
   Cotton is more "breathable" than synthetics, which helps offset the effects of a hot flash. Also, dress in layers that can be removed.

6. **Carry items that help you cool down quickly.**
   A portable, battery-operated fan and premoistened towelettes are both good choices for cooling down when a hot flash hits.

7. **Watch what you eat.**
   Eat plenty of fresh fruits and vegetables (at least five servings

daily) and use high-quality protein sources like soy foods and whole grains, emphasizing beans, legumes, raw nuts and seeds. Avoid sugary, fatty foods and meats, and remember that nutritional demands rise after menopause. Women who eat a vegetable-based diet suffer from fewer hormone-induced problems.

8. **Take a calcium/magnesium supplement, and drink at least 64 ounces of water daily.**

9. **Begin (or continue) a regular exercise program.**

Long-term aerobic and weight-bearing exercises prevent weight gain, osteoporosis, moodiness and other hormone- induced symptoms.

10. **Watch your blood sugar.**

Controlling blood sugar decreases the risk of heart disease and other health problems.

HOMEOPATHIC PREPARATIONS FOR HOT FLASHES

Homeopathic remedies are based on the "paradox rule," which claims that taking very tiny amounts of certain compounds that actually cause the ailment may work to alleviate it.

Belladonna. For sudden and intense hot flashes that may be accompanied by a throbbing headache, irritability and blood pressure changes.

Calcarea carbonica. For night sweats and flushing accompanied by weight gain, fatigue and stiff joints in the legs and feet.

Graphites. For hot flashes accompanied by mental sluggishness, weight gain and skin problems.

Ignatia. For hot flashes accompanied by dramatic mood swings, anxiety and muscle spasms.

Lachesis. For intense hot flashes accompanied by congestion and emotional problems.

Sepia. For hot flashes with by irregular periods and food cravings.

HOMEOPATHY DOSAGES

Use a lower potency (6X, 6C, 12X, 12C, 30X or 30C) or follow label directions. If no response is seen within a reasonable amount of time, select a different remedy.

The Natural Progesterone Phenomenon

By now, you've undoubtedly heard about the popularity of natural progesterone creams. Is there anything to these creams? Dr. John Lee is considered the ultimate guru of natural progesterone and is responsible for its emergence as a viable treatment for women. While more studies are needed, the logic behind using natural progesterone is compelling, to say the least.

Dr. Townsend believes that combining natural progesterone with the action of soy isoflavones provides women with powerful hormonal effects. The duo "covers all the bases" and works synergistically to address a number of female health problems, both pre and postmenopausal. A report in *Gynecological Endocrinology* states that using natural progesterone is appealing because it poses no risks to liver health, which is a major worry with prescription hormones. The value of natural progesterone is based on the very real phenomenon of estrogen dominance.

Estrogen excess or dominance can affect women of all ages but is most commonly seen in women in their forties. PMS, breast tenderness, mood swings, heavy bleeding, fibroids and weight gain are all symptoms of an estrogen overload. Women whose estrogen levels are not kept in check by the mitigating effects of progesterone can experience a myriad of symptoms and have a greater risk of developing breast or uterine cancer. Remember, however, that it doesn't matter whether you make a little or a lot of estrogen—if estrogen levels are not adequately balanced by progesterone, estrogen dominance can occur.

Unfortunately, many doctors will prescribe a synthetic estrogen drug to treat the symptoms listed on the following page (the worst thing they could do), when what most women really need is a safe and effective source of progesterone.

PROGESTERONE, NOT ESTROGEN, FOR MENOPAUSE

Evidence of depleted progesterone levels in women of all ages continues to mount. Until recently, however, most medical doctors have concentrated only on the fact that the estrogen levels of menopausal women dip. The role that a woman's disappearing progesterone plays has been neglected. Dr. Lee believes that problems associated with menopause are not caused by lack of estrogen, but by a lack of progesterone. He points out that while estrogen production drops to around 40 percent during menopause,

Symptoms of Estrogen Dominance

- weight gain (esp. hips and thighs)
- heavy menstrual flow or irregular periods
- carbohydrate cravings
- depression
- fatigue
- inability to focus
- thyroid dysfunction
- fibrocystic breasts
- uterine fibroids
- PMS
- loss of libido
- mood swings/depression
- certain types of acne
- breast enlargement/tenderness
- water retention
- endometriosis
- headaches
- hypoglycemia/blood sugar disorders
- uterine cramping
- infertility
- inability to maintain pregnancy
- cold hands and feet
- increased risk of endometrial (uterine) and breast cancers
- increased blood clotting, which raises the risk of stroke

progesterone production stops altogether, creating an estrogen dominance even in postmenopausal women. Keep in mind also that progesterone helps reduce the risk of breast and uterine cancer, while estrogen can stimulate the growth of malignant tumors in sensitive tissue.

Dr. Lee also points out that using synthetic estrogen drugs in menopausal women who make no progesterone is even more dangerous. Some studies have found that women who are low in progesterone are ten times more likely to die from cancer than those who have normal levels of the hormone.

PROGESTIN AND PROGESTERONE—SIMILAR IN NAME ONLY

Progesterone is produced in the ovaries and increases during the luteal phase (second portion) of the menstrual cycle. It dips down during the follicular phase (first portion) of the cycle and is also low before puberty. Production of progesterone stops altogether after menopause.

Progestin drugs are in no way, shape or form related to natural progesterone. Progestins are patented, synthetic drugs that are not well tolerated by the female body—as evidenced by their many side effects and health risks; whereas, unpatentable, natural progesterone is readily accepted by the body with few (or no) side effects or health risks. Natural progesterone has a different chemical structure than progestin. It effects the body through different pathways and is vital for normal uterine and breast development and to keep a pregnancy in place for nine months.

Although artificial progestins have been linked to cancer and heart disease, natural progesterone has shown a cancer-protective effect in breast tissue. Keep in mind that progestins can increase levels of LDL (bad) cholesterol and decrease HDL (good) cholesterol. In contrast, natural progesterone has no adverse effect on HDL cholesterol levels. Therefore, the best choice for treating conditions like PMS is natural progesterone rather than the progestins found in birth control pills and other synthetic hormones.

WHAT ABOUT WILD YAM?

Don't confuse natural progesterone with wild yam. Although many natural progesterone creams contain wild yam, they must be potentiated with additional natural USP progesterone to be effective. Wild yam contains a precursor compound to progesterone (diosgenin) that can be converted into progesterone in a laboratory. There has been some debate over whether wild yam is converted into progesterone in the body, but now the consensus is that it is unlikely. Wild yam alone has not been associated with a rise in progesterone levels in the body. Wild yam is considered a phytoestrogen, however, and also contains a variety of valuable compounds, so its use is not discouraged.

AVAILABLE FORMS OF NATURAL PROGESTERONE

Natural progesterone supplements come in pills, creams, lozenges, suppositories and in injectable forms. Natural progesterone creams containing USP progesterone are derived from the diosgenin found in Mexican wild yam and soybeans. Through a process that is carried out in a laboratory, diosgenin is chemically changed into a compound that is virtually identical to human progesterone.

Micronized progesterone has been produced in such a way that it can survive the digestive process when taken orally. It has been

Therapeutic Applications for Natural Progesterone

- enhances libido
- protects the uterus and breasts from malignancies (cancer)
- contributes to blood clotting
- is a precursor of corticosterones
- normalizes zinc and copper levels
- maintains the secretory endometrium
- is necessary for the survival and development of the fetus
- helps to prevent osteoporosis
- is needed for the proper production of adrenal hormones
- works to stabilize blood sugar
- has a natural diuretic action
- prevents salt retention
- acts as an antidepressant
- helps to prevent the formation of fibrocystic breasts
- enhances thermogenesis (the burning of fat)
- contributes to the regulation of the thyroid gland

shown to improve menopausal symptoms but is available only by prescription. This is the only oral form of progesterone that survives the digestive process. This alternative to cream formulations may help to treat hot flashes, mood slumps, irritability, insomnia and sexual dysfunction. Because it is relatively new, more data is needed to assess its full value.

NATURAL PROGESTERONE DOSAGES

Look for natural progesterone creams that contain USP progesterone, and use enough cream to deliver between 15 and 20 milligrams of progesterone daily. Dr. Lee recommends using 15 to 24 milligrams per day for fourteen days before your expected period if you are a premenopausal woman and 15 milligrams per day for twenty-five days of the calendar month for postmenopausal women.

The cream should be applied where the skin is the thinnest and where multiple veins are visible. I have found that the wrist, the back of the hand, and breast tissue are the best areas for maximal absorption. The thighs and abdominal wall are poor receptor sites because the skin is tougher, thicker and has more layers of fat with few visible blood vessels. Approximately one half teaspoon of a progesterone cream used daily should provide around 20 milligrams.

NATURAL PROGESTERONE: SAFETY ISSUES

Natural progesterone is considered safe. To date, combining it with other drugs has not resulted in any interference or alteration. Its safety for pregnant or nursing mothers, however, has not been clinically documented. If you want a personal progesterone profile, Dr. Lee suggests a saliva test, which he considers more accurate than traditional blood tests.

How to Prevent and Even Reverse Bone Loss

The threat of developing osteoporosis is another reason why women take HRT. Osteoporosis causes bones to become brittle raising the risk of bone fracture (especially in the hip, spine and wrist). Although the disease runs in families, any woman with low estrogen levels may also begin to lose bone mass.

WHEN DOES BONE LOSS START?

You don't have to be menopausal to start losing bone density. In fact, by the time you get to menopause, you may have already lost considerable bone mass. Poor bone health can start in the early years. Unquestionably, young women do not consume sufficient amounts of calcium to maintain good bone density. This lack of calcium coupled with stress, dieting, eating disorders, lack of ovulation and lack of exercise can predispose these women to brittle bones.

RISK FACTORS THAT RAISE YOUR RISK OF OSTEOPOROSIS

1. Ovarian failure.

Young women who fail to menstruate but are not pregnant may develop something called "premature ovarian failure." This condition indicates that their hormonal output is not sufficient to drive a normal cycle. When a woman's ovaries cease production of hormones prior to age thirty-five, bone loss can accelerate. According to the National Institutes of Health (NIH), roughly 1 percent of American women experience ovarian failure by age forty. (This could be the subject of a book all by itself.) Granted, no woman is going to complain if she is spared a period or two; however, missing periods should not be taken lightly. You should see your doctor and ask to have your hormone levels checked for ovarian failure.

2. Using birth control pills.

In light of the above information, it only stands to reason that women who are taking birth control pills have lower bone mineral density (BMD) than women who have never used oral contraceptives. Studies indicate that their bone mineral density was 2.3 percent to 3.7 percent lower than women who did not use the pill.

3. High salt intake.

While we still need more data, it is clear that consuming salt in the short term resulted in more calcium loss in the urine. The higher the calcium count of the urine—the higher the risk of bone loss. As mentioned, a conclusive and supported link between salt intake and osteoporosis has not yet been established, but common sense says that cutting down on salt is a smart move.

4. Consuming carbonated drinks and caffeine.

Drinking soda pop may also raise your risk for osteoporosis. Many of these beverages contain phosphoric acid, which is thought to leech calcium from the bones. In one study, children who drank six glasses of these soft drinks had more than five times the risk of developing low blood levels of calcium compared with other children. Keep in mind, that most soda pop also contains sodium, which may also weaken bone strength. Caffeine intake also results in more calcium loss in the urine. Women who consume caffeine appear to have a higher risk of hip fractures and also have lower-than-normal bone mass.

5. Consuming detrimental dairy.

Why are women who live in England, Australia and the United States the most prone to osteoporosis when they are the same women who consume the most dairy products? Although dairy products are typically high in calcium, there are theories which suggest that the calcium content of processed cheeses and pasteurized milk is not adequately absorbed into the bones and teeth. In addition, eating large amounts of red meat combined with dairy may also negatively impact bone mass. Look for dairy products that are high in calcium and low in fat and salt. Many active-culture yogurts are good choices.

6. Smoking and using prescription drugs.

Smoking most definitely causes increased bone loss, not to mention a whole host of other terrible health problems. In addition drugs likes synthroid (used to treat hypothyroidism or an underactive thyroid) weakens bones. If you take this drug, supplementing your diet with absorbable forms of calcium (calcium citrate, gluconate, etc.) is vital.

DRUGS FOR OSTEOPOROSIS

Conventional treatment options for osteoporosis include prescription drugs that suppress the breakdown of bone (e.g., alendronate [Fosamax], calcitonin [Calcimir, Miacalcin], raloxifene [Evista]), as well as those that provide hormone replacement therapy (e.g., estradiol [Estrace, Estraderm, Fempatch], conjugated estrogens [Premarin], and conjugated estrogens with medroxyprogesterone acetate [Premphase, Prempro, Provera]) for postmenopausal women. Many of these drugs come with unpleasant side effects that should be discussed thoroughly with your doctor. Thankfully, Mother Nature provides viable alternatives that are infinitely safer.

DOES HRT PREVENT OSTEOPOROSIS?

Women in western societies generally eat lots of dairy and take HRT but still have a massive problem with bone loss. Yet women in third world countries, who eat virtually no dairy or meat, generally escape osteoporosis. Of equal importance, these women certainly don't use HRT after menopause, so how do they avoid the bone pitfalls of disappearing estrogen?

There is enough research data to question the effectiveness of synthetic hormones for preventing bone loss. Do the pros outweigh the cons? It's doubtful. The ability of estrogen to prevent osteoporosis is still being debated, but we do know that HRT cannot increase bone mass or replace bone tissue.

BONE DENSITY AND SOY ISOFLAVONES

Research out of the University of Illinois in Urbana tells us that soy isoflavones can help to strengthen the bones of the lumbar spine. When patients consumed 92 milligrams of soy isoflavones per day, bone density increased by 2.2 percent over a period of six months. Keep in mind that the majority of women lose 2 to 3 percent of bone density in the two to three years following menopause. What this suggests is that the sooner we increase our intake of isoflavones, the better it is for our bones.

EAT MORE SOY FOODS

Look to tofu, soy milk, roasted soy beans and soy protein powders to protect bones. Soy isoflavones have been shown to protect against bone loss in several animal studies. In a double-blind trial, postmenopausal women who supplemented their diet with 40 grams of soy protein powder (containing 90 milligrams of isoflavones) per day were protected against bone mineral loss in the spine, although lower amounts of soy were not protective.

IPRIFLAVONE: POTENTIATED BONE-PROTECTIVE ISOFLAVONE

In 1988, Japan registered an osteoporosis drug called Ipriflavone. Simply put, it is a synthetic flavonoid compound produced from daidzein (another soy isoflavone). European and Japanese practitioners use Ipriflavone to treat bone loss, and it is now available as a dietary supplement. It appears to increase the activity of bone-building cells called *osteoblasts*, while simultaneously inhibiting the action of osteoclasts (which break down bone tissue).

Of equal (or more) importance is the result of a recent study showing that Ipriflavone dramatically boosted new bone formation and repair. Fifty-six postmenopausal women with low bone density received 1,000 milligrams of calcium, and random subjects were given an additional 600 milligrams of Ipriflavone. The women who took only the calcium actually experienced increased bone loss after two years. By contrast, bone loss was totally halted in those who took the Ipriflavone. Researchers concluded that "Ipriflavone prevents the rapid bone loss following early menopause." How does it work? While it does not exert an estrogenic effect in the body, it does boost estrogen action in the body. The recommended dosage of Ipriflavone is 600 milligrams daily.

NATURAL PROGESTERONE INCREASES BONE MASS

Without question, natural progesterone cream should be included in any regimen to prevent osteoporosis. Dr. John Lee has documented his experiences with scores of women who suffered from osteoporosis and continually lost bone mass. Many of them were on estrogen replacement therapy. While he concedes that estrogen therapy may have slowed their bone loss, it did nothing to reverse the disease. Even when these women took calcium, vitamins D and C and even quit smoking, their bone loss continued.

Dr. Lee states that over a three-year period most women who did not take HRT lost 4.5 percent of their bone mass. He found that by adding natural progesterone treatments, these women experienced a 15 percent increase in bone mass over a period of three years with no negative side effects.

CHOOSE CALCIUM

All calcium supplements are not created equal, and research shows that not all supplements contain comparable amounts of elemental calcium (nor are they absorbed in the same way). Calcium citrate is a good choice. Take 1,200 to 1,500 milligrams prior to retiring. Don't take it with fiber, however, or its absorption will be impaired. Moreover, do not use oyster shells, dolomite or bone meal as sources of calcium. They can contain lead or other toxins.

If it's not included in your calcium supplement, add magnesium and vitamin D. Magnesium supplementation at 250 to 750 milligrams per day has been shown to stop bone loss while boosting bone mass in 87 percent of people with osteoporosis in a two-year, controlled trial. Take at least 350 milligrams of magnesium daily. And remember that a deficiency of vitamin D is common in the elderly and can speed up bone loss. Studies show that vitamin D supplementation in particular reduces bone loss in women who don't get it through their diet. You should be taking 800 IU per day with your calcium for maximum benefit. If possible, start supplementing when you are young.

GOOD FATS ARE WHERE IT'S AT

One study revealed that older women with osteoporosis who were given 4 grams of fish oil per day for four months had improved calcium absorption and even showed evidence of new bone formation. Combing fish oil with evening primrose oil (EPO) may render even better results. In another study, women who took 6 grams of a combination of EPO and fish oil plus 600 mg of calcium per day for three years experienced no spinal bone loss in the first eighteen months and showed a dramatic 3.1 percent increase in spinal bone mineral density during the last eighteen months.

THE BONE-BOOSTING GAME PLAN

Eat more soy. Soy isoflavones work to protect bone mass.

Use a natural progesterone cream. Natural progesterone may even reverse bone loss.

Eat more vegetables. A diet rich in vegetables helps to keep your blood more alkaline, which can prevent mineral depletion from the bones. They are also rich in vitamin K, which works to maintain calcium deep within your bones.

Take a calcium supplement. If women began to take good calcium supplements early in life, millions of dollars could be saved on medical care required to treat bone fractures of the elderly.

Magnify your magnesium. Low blood and bone levels of magnesium have been found in women with osteoporosis.

Choose your oils wisely. Consume coldwater fish (tuna, salmon, etc.) on a regular basis, or take essential fatty acid supplements that contain EPA, DHA and omega-3 fatty acids.

Vitamin K keeps bones healthy. Along with calcium, magnesium and vitamin D, women who have osteoporosis often have low levels of vitamin K. One study found that postmenopausal women can decrease loss of calcium in the urine by taking 1 milligram of vitamin K per day. And those who already had osteoporosis and took 45 milligrams of vitamin K per day showed an increase in bone density after six months and an overall decreased bone loss.

Minerals for bone mass. Trace minerals like zinc and copper are also vital for bone mass production and should be part of a daily supplement program. Take 10 milligrams of zinc and 2 to 3 milligrams of copper daily.

Engage in weight-bearing exercise. Weight-bearing exercises can do wonders for bone strength and can be combined with aerobic exercises like walking. Studies indicate that women who exercise at least three times a week have a higher bone mineral content.

Using weights can also be beneficial, but you should avoid any maneuver that puts too much stress on your bones and joints.

Hormone-Friendly Herbs

IMPRESSIVE PLANT ESTROGENS

Several herbs contain "phyto" or plant estrogens. These compounds have chemical structures that mimic human estrogen in the female body. In fact, these remarkable compounds have biochemical "smarts." In premenopausal women they block high estrogen levels, while in aging women they boost estrogenic actions. These user-friendly compounds (called *isoflavones*) give a plant its estrogenic action. Researchers at the Department of Obstetrics and Gynecology at the University of Bari, Italy, have concluded that phytoestrogens increase bone density and reduce cholesterol. They believe that the estrogenic effects of phytoestrogens may be useful in preventing postmenopausal cardiovascular disease as well as osteoporosis. We've talked about soy phytoestrogens called isoflavones. An herb called red clover is also chock-full of them.

RED CLOVER

Known for its sweet-scented and round, purplish blossoms, red clover grows in meadows and near roadsides all over the world. Steeped in lore and legend, some once believed that carrying a red clover would attract the company of good fairies. For a millennia, Chinese and Russian health practitioners have prescribed red clover tea for everything from asthma and kidney stones to psoriasis. During the 1930s, red clover was part of the famous Hoxsey Formula, an herbal regimen for treating cancer.

Current interest in the herb centers on its role as a phytoestrogen for hormonal dysfunction. The fact that red clover has been successfully used in Australia (Promensel) for a number of gynecological problems has sparked new interest in the dainty, fragrant plant for women in this country.

Red Clover Is Rich in Isoflavones

While soy is best known for two isoflavones (genistein and daidzein), red clover contains all four (formononetin, genistein, daidzein and biochanin). The isoflavone content of red clover is concentrated, so a little red clover goes a long way. For women who have trouble eating enough soy to get the isoflavone count they need, a red clover supplement may be the solution. If your menstrual cycles are coming to an end, it holds particular promise.

Clover Clobbers "The Change"

Deborah Gordon, M.D., author of *Menopause the Natural Way*, recommends red clover for the hot flashes, insomnia and mood slumps that can accompany menopause. Dr. Gordon cites a double-blind study of eighty-six perimenopausal women who were given a red clover supplement containing 40 milligrams of isoflavones (per 500 milligram tablet). Doctors recorded symptoms for eight months and found a high correlation between the intake of isoflavones from red clover and a reduction in hot flashes.

Red Clover for Women's Heart Health

As mentioned earlier, one major health risk of menopause is heart disease. Cardiovascular disease is the leading killer of women over age forty-five, and one reason doctors strongly advised using HRT in the past (though we know better now). In 1998, news wires reported the successful use of a compound extracted from red clover called P-081 to significantly increase HDL (good) cholesterol levels in a group of postmenopausal women. Dr. Rodney J. Barber, a gynecologist from Sydney, Australia, presented these findings at the 10th annual meeting of the North American Menopause Society. The study included fifty women, aged fifty to sixty-four. Those women who received a 50 milligram dose of the supplement over a period of several weeks saw a rise in their HDL cholesterol levels by an average of 28.6 percent. (More HDLs mean better heart protection.)

Another controlled trial published in the March 1999 issue of the *Journal of Clinical Endocrinology and Metabolism* showed that red clover isoflavones help keep large blood vessels pliable—something that could prevent heart disease. In a placebo-controlled trial, women who received 80 milligrams of isoflavones derived from red clover improved the elasticity of their arteries by 23 percent.

Red Clover for Endometriosis and Menstrual Woes

Michael Murray, N.D., author of *The Encyclopedia of Natural Medicine*, says "One of the most common findings in women with PMS (premenstrual syndrome) is an elevated estrogen-to-progesterone ratio." When estrogen is not properly balanced with progesterone, it stimulates a variety of feminine foibles (i.e. bloating, tender breasts, cramps, heavy menstrual flow, and fibroids) typically associated with PMS. Murray stresses that phytoestrogens exert a "balancing action" on estrogen. How? The isoflavones found in red clover bump potent estrogens off of receptors cells, replacing them with a gentler, kinder version; hence, estrogen-driven symptoms typically seen in PMS are reduced, and estrogen/progesterone ratios fall into better equilibrium.

The growth of endometrial tissue is also stimulated by the presence of estrogen. Most drugs designed to treat endometriosis are strong estrogen blockers. Taking red clover prompts the body to excrete more estrogen. When the plant's much weaker form binds to receptor sites, human estrogen has nowhere to go so it is eliminated in the urine. Less circulating estrogen means less endometrial growth and cramping.

Boosting Breast Health

Red clover can produce the same beneficial effect in the breasts. Fibrocystic breast disease occurs in approximately 80 percent of premenopausal women and can be stimulated by estrogen overload. Because the phytoestrogens found in red clover attach to breast tissue instead of other estrogens, the growth of benign cysts is limited. James Marti, author of *The Alternative Health & Medicine Encyclopedia*, points out that herbs like red clover have shown some success in treating fibrocystic breast disease.

When it comes to breast cancer, dozens of studies show that phytoestrogens actually inhibit breast cancer cell growth. A study published in the November 1990 issue of *Oncology Report* stated that phytoestrogens—genistein, daidzein, biochanin A and coumestrol (all of which are found in red clover)—inhibited laboratory-stimulated tumor growth in breast cancer cells.

Red Clover Dosage Recommendations

Red clover is available in various forms: dried bulk, capsules, tinctures and teas. Medical herbalist, Tammi Hartung, author of *Growing Herbs That Heal*, suggests adding it to rice, salads and other dishes, as well as using it in supplement form. Take two 500 milligram capsules three times daily, at mealtimes. Red clover tea can be made by adding one to three teaspoons of the dried herb to a cup of boiling water and steeping the tea for ten to fifteen minutes (taken three times daily). Keep in mind that it is more difficult to know how many isoflavones you actually get from teas. You may not see any noticeable difference until you've been on the supplement for three to six weeks, and if you stop, the benefits will cease.

Red Clover Caveats

People on blood-thinning drugs such as Coumadin (warfarin) should not take red clover because of the naturally occurring salicylates in the plant that are natural anticoagulants. Pregnant or nursing women should not use red clover, and it is not for children under ten years of age. No interactions have been reported from combining standard HRT or oral contraceptives with red clover, but check with your health care provider as a precaution. If you have had breast cancer or are undergoing treatment, check with your doctor before taking any supplement.

OTHER PHYTOESTROGENIC HERBS

Black Cohosh Root

Black cohosh also contains phytoestrogens that may have value for menopausal disorders and premenstrual complaints. Black cohosh is used extensively in Europe and has received official recognition as a supplement in Great Britain and Germany. Studies have shown that black cohosh root has endocrine activity similar to soy isoflavones. It's antispasmodic and diuretic actions also contribute to the herb's usefulness for cramping and other symptoms of PMS. It is typically used to treat hot flashes, vaginal dryness and depression associated with menopause. Take 2 to 4 milligrams of the extract (also called *Cimicifuga racemosa*) or as directed. This herb should not be used by pregnant or nursing women or in large doses.

Dong Quai

Used extensively by Chinese practitioners for the treatment of gynecological ailments, dong quai may have value for several symptoms of menopause. Dong quai is believed to have analgesic properties, which are probably due in part to its antispasmodic effect. It also boosts elimination, acts as a natural estrogen and supports the cardiovascular system—all very beneficial effects for menopausal women. Take one-fourth teaspoon of an extract daily. This herb should not be used by pregnant or nursing women or by anyone with hemorrhagic disease. Dong quai should also be avoided during severe cases of influenza. Exposure to the sun while taking this herb may cause rash or aggravated sunburn in some people.

Chaste Berry (Vitex)

Vitex acts on the pituitary gland to normalize hormonal function, and substantial clinical evidence bears out its value for PMS, menopausal complaints and even infertility. A team of German investigators conducted a controlled, double-blind study to evaluate the efficacy and safety of a standardized vitex supplement in comparison with pyridoxine (vitamin B6) in 175 women with PMS. Vitex was associated with considerably better relief of typical PMS complaints, such as breast tenderness, edema, tension, headache, constipation and depression. Use a standardized vitex product that contains 0.5 agnuside and take 175 to 225 milligrams daily.

Licorice Root

Another favorite herb of Chinese practitioners, licorice root is used in about one-third of all Chinese herbal formulas and is widely used for female disorders. Licorice root controls water retention, breast tenderness, carbohydrate cravings and other symptoms of hormone fluctuation by helping to balance hormones.

Use only DGL (deglycyrrhizinated) licorice products and take 250 to 500 milligrams daily. People with high blood pressure, heart arrhythmias, or kidney disease should avoid it, as well as anyone on digoxin-based drugs or digitalis—unless supervised by a physician. Taking licorice for long periods of time can raise blood pressure. Taking potassium supplements with licorice root is advised.

Gotu Kola, Ginkgo and St. John's Wort

These herbs help to boost brain function and fight the mood changes, irritability, lack of focus and depression that can accompany PMS or menopause. Take as directed using standardized products or guaranteed potency products.

VITAMINS AND MINERALS FOR HORMONE BALANCE

Vitamin B-Complex

Some research indicates that B-complex vitamins protect against some of the dangerous effects of estradiol and estrone in the body. Moreover, estrogen imbalances have been linked to a vitamin B6 deficiency. Several clinical trials show that B vitamins can also help ease the symptoms of PMS and fight depression and stress. Take as directed using a B25 or B50 formula. Taking extra vitamin B6 may also be helpful. This vitamin specifically treats water retention and helps to fight mood swings that can occur during PMS or menopause.

Vitamin E

Studies reveal that vitamin E supplements dramatically impact hot flashes and other menopausal symptoms. In some tests, vitamin E calmed anxiety better than barbituates. While some data surrounding the use of vitamin E and breast cancer is controversial, the overwhelming consensus is that this vitamin helps to prevent breast fibroids, reduces the risk of heart disease and may help to ease hormone- induced symptoms. Take 200 to 400 IU daily of natural products.

Vitamin C with Hesperidin

In a recent clinical study of ninety-four menopausal women, researchers found that using vitamin C with hesperidin (a bioflavonoid) relieved symptoms in 50 percent of participants. Leg cramps, bruising and hot flashes also decreased significantly. Some bioflavonoids actually resemble estradiol in their chemical structure. Take 500 to 1,000 milligrams daily.

Calcium/Magnesium

These two minerals help to calm anxiety by quieting the central nervous system. Calcium and magnesium also provide a buffer against bone loss, which threatens some women after menopause when drops in estrogen increase the risk of osteoporosis. Take 1,500 milligrams of calcium citrate and 1,000 milligrams of chelated magnesium daily.

Vitamin D

Many postmenopausal women have impaired synthesis of vitamin D, which inhibits the absorption of calcium. One cause of this may be reduced exposure to sun. When you are out in the sun, your skin naturally produces vitamin D. Older women who don't expose their skin to sunlight may find themselves with a vitamin D deficiency. Supplements may be the answer. Women who are unable to get outside much should supplement their diet with 400 to 800 IU daily.

OTHER NATURAL COMPOUNDS FOR HORMONE- DRIVEN SYMPTOMS

Quercitin and Curcumin

Studies have found that adding curcumin (found in turmeric root) to genistein (a soy isoflavone) greatly boosted its anti-estrogenic effects. In one study, curcumin and genistein worked together synergistically to inhibit the growth of human breast cancer cells created by exposure to powerful estrogenic pesticides. Scientists concluded the combination of curcumin and genistein in the diet may prevent hormone-related cancers stimulated by our environment. Quercitin, a bioflavonoid and powerful antioxidant, has a similar effect. Take 500 milligrams of quercitin and 600 milligrams of curcumin daily.

Gamma-Oryzanol

This compound is extracted from rice bran and can help to modulate hot flashes and other menopausal symptoms. Take 20 milligrams daily.

5-Hydroxytryptophan (5-HTP)

Some clinical trials reveal that low blood levels of tryptophan and estrogen were found in women who suffered from depression during menopause. Moreover, 5-HTP may help promote more restful sleep which can be impaired during menopause. An article in the *Journal of Psychiatry and Neuroscience* stated that supplemental tryptophan also reduced several symptoms of PMS including insomnia, irritability and carbohydrate cravings. Take 100 to 200 milligrams three times daily.

Superior Female Health Naturally: The Game Plan

1. Add soy to your diet.

By using soy powders, tofu, soy milk, soy nuts, etc., you should be able to consume no less than 25 and no more than 60 grams of soy protein (and approximately 35 milligrams of isoflavones) daily. One or two servings of tofu, soybeans or soy milk a day is equivalent to the typical soy intake of most Asian women. One cup of soybeans provides 300 milligrams of isoflavones. If you are not going to consistently consume soy foods on a daily basis, consider a soy or genistein supplement. If you are allergic to soy, red clover supplementation is an option. Black cohosh, dong quai and vitex are also options for women with soy allergies.

2. Use natural progesterone.

Using an effective natural progesterone cream can oppose estrogen in a safe way when you're not pregnant. You may have noticed from early discussions about progesterone in this booklet that many of its actions are just the opposite of estrogen-driven symptoms.

3. Eat plenty of cruciferous vegetables.

Cruciferous vegetables are those with four-petal flowers resembling a cross, including arugula, bok choy, broccoli, broccoli sprouts, Brussels sprouts, cabbage, cauliflower, Swiss chard, collards, kale, kohlrabi, mustard greens, radishes, rutabaga, turnips, turnip greens and watercress. The typical Asian diet is not only high in soy but in cabbage consumption as well, suggesting that the combination of cruciferous vegetables with soy makes for a healthy duo.

One phytochemical, indole-3-carbinol, has already accrued some impressive data backing its use as an effective estrogen blocker. In a study at the Institute for Hormone Research in New York, twelve healthy volunteers (seven men and five women) were given daily doses of 350 to 500 milligrams of indole-3-carbinol (I3C), which is equivalent to 10 to 12 ounces of raw cabbage or Brussels sprouts. After a week, indole-3-carbinol had converted estrogen into a metabolite other than the one linked to the formation of cancer. This effect was later duplicated using a cruciferous vegetable extract in a larger group of women. If you are not going to eat these veggies, consider using an indole-3-carbinol supplement at 300 to 600 milligrams per day.

4. Be picky about your fats.

Limit omega-6 fats (i.e. corn, cottonseed oil, peanut and grape-seed oils) and increase your intake of omega-3 fats (found in fish oils). (Both are types of polyunsaturated fat.) A study published in a leading medical journal found that using omega-6 polyunsaturated fat increased the risk of breast cancer by almost 70 percent.

Eating fish on a regular basis is a great way to get omega-3 fatty acids. If you're not a fish eater, use a supplement. Taking flaxseed oil daily is another way to get the essential fatty acids you need. Flaxseed oil may lower the production of potentially dangerous estrogens by blocking some of their tumor-initiating effects. A 1993 article published in *Clinical Endocrinology Metabolism* found that flaxseed enhances progesterone/estradiol ratios during menstruation. It can be taken as a supplement or can be used as the oil in salads, etc. You should take approximately 30 grams of flaxseed oil per day, especially if you are allergic to soy foods. You may also want to use olive oil for cooking and salad dressings. Olive oil, a monounsaturated fat, may actually protect breast tissue against the formation of cancerous tumors.

Avoid saturated fats found in dairy and animal foods. Solid margarines and shortenings may also contain dangerous trans-fatty acids, which are created when liquid oil is converted to a solid. These artificial fat compounds have been linked with increased artery disease as well as breast cancer. Avoid hydrogenated or partially hydrogenated fats, which hides in many cookies, crackers, muffins, pies, etc.

5. Fiber, fiber, fiber.

Get fiber! Studies reveal that estrogen levels go down when sufficient amounts of wheat bran are added to a woman's diet. The insoluble fiber found in this kind of bran actually binds to estrogen in the bowel, boosting its elimination. If waste estrogen sits in the colon too long, it can be reabsorbed back into the blood stream. Fiber-full diets help to prevent this phenomenon. (And remember that if you take synthetic estrogens, fiber will affect the way these hormones will be metabolized in your liver.)

Beans are full of fiber, as are whole grains, fruit peelings and veggies. If you have a problem with constipation, fix it. Taking magnesium in combination with herbs like *Cascara sagrada* can initiate bowel movements without cramping or addiction. Psyllium hulls contained in laxatives like Metamucil are also effective. Eat foods rich in fiber such as beans, sprouts, whole grains, almonds, sunflower seed, lentils, split peas, parsley, blueberries, endive, oats, potatoes (with skin), carrots and peaches . Eat insoluble fiber—like wheat and oat bran—on a daily basis as well.

6. Remember the sugar link to hormones.

Lowering your blood sugar and insulin levels can help ease estrogen excess. Some studies have shown that women with high insulin levels have a dramatically higher risk of developing breast cancer. Keep in mind that the more sugar and starch you eat, the more insulin is secreted into the bloodstream. It is also thought that insulin may stimulate the growth of estrogen-dependent cancers. In fact, a report in the *American Journal of Obstetrics and Gynecology* points out that synthetic hormones found in HRT have an adverse effect on insulin resistance. According to an article in a 1991 issue of the *Journal of Reproductive Medicine*, the consumption of foods and beverages high in sugar is associated with the prevalence of PMS. Avoid refined sugars, white flour and foods that have a high glycemic rating (they convert to glucose very quickly).

7. Move your body!

Hot flashes are half as common in women who engage in regular physical activity compared with those who don't. Exercise is a win-win proposition. Not only does exercise help keep fat stores down (fat cells make estrogen), it also chases the blues away, de-stresses the body and mind, and keeps the heart and bones healthy. What better prescription for hormone- driven disorders and menopause? Regular exercise may be a woman's best defense against these symptoms.

Participate in an aerobic workout (brisk walking, jogging, biking, etc.) three to five times a week for thirty-five to forty-five minutes daily. Working out with weights is also good to build muscle mass and prevent osteoporosis. The important thing is to start slowly and build up. And always check with your doctor before starting an exercise program.

References

Adams, M.R., Register, T.C., Golden, D.L., et al. "Medroxyprogesterone acetate antagonizes inhibitory effects of conjugated equine estrogens on coronary artery atherosclerosis." *Arteriosclerosis and Thrombocitic and Vascular Biology.* 1997: (17)217–21.

"A dietary supplement derived from red clover, called P-081, significantly increased HDL ('good') cholesterol levels in postmenopausal women, according to results of a study." *Reuters Health.* 1998, Sept 27.

Albertazzi, P. "Purified phytoestrogens in postmenopausal bone health: is there a role for genistein?" *Climacteric.* 2002, June 5: (2)190–196.

"American Heart Association President Robert Bonow, M.D., Responds to New Findings from Women's Health Initiative Trial." 2002, July 9. Media advisory. americanheart.org.

Bahl, V.K. and N. Naik. "Hormone replacement therapy and coronary artery disease: buried alive?" *Indian Heart J.* 2001 Nov-Dec: 53(6):707-13.

Berger, D., Schaffner, W., Schrader, E., et al. "Efficacy of *Vitex agnus castus* L. extract Ze 440 in patients with premenstrual syndrome (PMS)." *Archival Gynecology and Obstetrics.* 2000, Nov: 264(3)150–3.

Blond, B. "Definitive contra-indications for menopausal hormone replacement therapy." *Soins.* 2001, Mar: (653)10.

Bravata, D.M., Rastegar, A. and R.I. Horwitz. "How do women make decisions about hormone replacement therapy?" *American Journal of Medicine.* 2002, Jul: 113(1)22–29.

Cangiano, C., et al. "Effects of oral 5-hydroxy-tryptophan on energy intake and macronutrient selection in non-insulin dependent diabetic patients." *International Journal of Obesity and Related Metabolic Disorders.* 1998, Jul: 22(7)648–654.

Carroll, D.G. and S.L. Noble. "Hormone replacement therapy: current concerns and considerations." *American Journal of Managed Care.* 2002, Jul: 8(7)663–675.

Chiechi, L.M. "Dietary phytoestrogens in the prevention of long-term postmenopausal diseases." Department of Obstetrics and Gynaecology III, University of Bari, Italy. *International Journal of Gynaecology and Obstetrics.* 1999, Oct: 67(1)39–40.

Cooper, A., Spencer, C., Whitehead, M.I., et al. "Systemic absorption of progesterone from Progest cream in postmenopausal women." *Lancet.* 1998: (351)1255–1256.

Cowan, L.D., Gordis, L., Tonascia, J.A. and G.S. Jones. "Breast cancer incidence in women with a history of progesterone deficiency." *American Journal of Epidemiology.* 1981: (114)209–217.

De Rijke, E., Zafra-Gomez, A., Ariese, F., Brinkman, U.A., et al. "Determination of isoflavone glucoside malonates in *Trifolium pratense* L. (red clover) extracts: quantification and stability studies." *Journal of Chromatography.* 2001, Oct 12: 932(1–2)55–64.

De Souza, M., et al. "A synergistic effect of a daily supplement for 1 month of 200 mg magnesium puls 50 mg vitamin B6 for the relief of anxiety-related premenstrual symptoms: a randomized, double-blind, crossover study." *Journal of Women's Health Gender Based Medicine.* 2000, Mar: 9(2)131–139.

Dixon, R.A. and D. Ferreira. "Genistein." *Phytochemistry.* 2002 Jun: 60(3)205–211.

Dixon-Shanies, D. and N. Shaikh. "Growth inhibition of human breast cancer cells by herbs and phytoestrogens." *Oncology Reports.* 1999, Nov-Dec: 6(6)1383–1387.

Dornstauder, E., Jisa, E., Unterrieder, I., et al. "Estrogenic activity of two standardized red clover extracts (Menoflavon) intended for large scale use in hormone replacement therapy." *J Steroid Biochemistry and Molecular Biology.* 2001, Jul: 78(1)67–75.

Eichholz, A.C., Mahavni, V. and A.K. Sood. "Allopathic and complementary alternatives to hormone replacement therapy." *Expert Opinions on Pharmacotherapy.* 2002, Jul: 3(7)949–955.

Emons, G. and S. Westphalen. "Hormone replacement therapy in peri- and postmenopause. Routine use is not indicated." *MMW Fortschr Med.* 2002, Feb 28: 144(9)30–33. German.

Enriori, P.J., Hirsig, R.J., Vico, C.M., et al. "Effect of natural 'micronized' progesterone on the chorionic gonadotropin concentrations in cyst fluids of women with gross cystic breast disease." *J Steroid Biochem Mol Biol.* 2000 May: 73(1-2):67-70.

Fritz, W.A., Wang, J., Eltoum, I.E., et al. "Dietary genistein down-regulates androgen and estrogen receptor expression in the rat prostate." *Molecular and Cellular Endocrinology.* 2002, Jan 15: 186(1)89–99.

Fugh-Berman, A., Kronenberg, F. "Red clover (*Trifolium pratense*) for menopausal women: current state of knowledge." *Menopause.* 2001, Sep–Oct: 8(5)333–337.

Gennari, C., Agnusdei, D., Crepaldi, G., et al. "Effect of ipriflavone—a synthetic derivative of natural isoflavones—on bone mass loss in the early years after menopause." *Menopause.* 1998, Spring: 5(1)9–15.

Gordon, Deborah, M.D. *Menopause The Natural Way.* (John Wiley & Sons, 2001).

Gupta, Sanjay. "Should anyone take hormones? A new study raises disturbing questions about the safety of hormone-replacement therapy." *Time.* 2002, Jul 15: 160(3)70.

Hale, G.E., Hughes, C.L., Robboy, S.J., et al. "A double-blind randomized study on the effects of red clover isoflavones on the endometrium." *Menopause.* 2001, Sep–Oct: 8(5)338–346.

Hargrove, J.T., Maxson, W.S., Wentz, A.C., et al. "Menopausal hormone replacement therapy with continuous daily oral micronized estradiol and progesterone." *Obstetrics and Gynecology.* 1989: (73)606–612.

Hargrove, J.T. and K.G. Osteen. "An alternative method of hormone replacement therapy using the natural sex steroids." *Infertility and Reproductive Medicine Clinic of North America.* 1995: (6)653–674.

Howes, J.B., Sullivan, D., Lai, N., et al. "The effects of dietary supplementation with isoflavones from red clover on the lipoprotein profiles of post menopausal women with mild to moderate hypercholesterolaemia." *Atherosclerosis.* 2000, Sept: 152(1)143–147.

Indian Heart Journal. 2002, Jan–Feb: 54(1)23–30.

Journal of Steroid Biochemistry and Molecular Biology. 2000, May: 73(1–2)67–70.

Journal of the American Medical Association. 2002, Jul 3: 288(1)99–101.

Journal of the Association of the Physicians of India. 2001, Dec: (49)1176–1180.

Lark, Susan, M.D. *PMS Premenstrual Syndrome Self Help Book.* (Celestial Arts, Berkeley: 1997).

Lee, J.R. "Osteoporosis reversal: the role of progesterone." *International Clinical Nutrition Review.* 1990: (10)384–391.

Leonetti, H.B., Longo, S. and J.M. Anasti. "Transdermal progesterone cream for vasomotor symptoms and postmenopausal bone loss." *Obstetrics and Gynecology.* 1999: (94)225–228.

Lieberman, S. "A review of the effectiveness of *Cimicifuga racemosa* (black cohosh) for the symptoms of menopause." *Journal of Womens Health.* 1998, Jun: 7(5)525–529.

Liu, J. "Natural progesterone." *Health News.* 1998, Mar 31: 4(4)3.

Liu, Z., Yang, Z., Zhu, M. and J. Huo. "Estrogenicity of black cohosh (*Cimicifuga racemosa*) and its effect on estrogen receptor level in human breast cancer MCF-7 cells." *Wei Sheng Yan Jiu.* 2001, Mar 30: (2)77–80.

Loch, E.G., Selle, H. and N. Boblitz. "Treatment of premenstrual syndrome with a phytopharmaceutical formulation containing *Vitex agnus castus*." *Journal of Womens Health and Gender Based Medicine.* 2000 Apr: 9(3)315–320.

Martorano, J.T., Ahlgrimm, M. and T. Colbert. "Differentiating between natural progesterone and synthetic progestins: clinical implications for premenstrual syndrome and perimenopause management." *Comprehensive Therapies.* 1998: (24)336–339.

McKenna, D.J., Jones, K., Humphrey, S., et al. "Black cohosh: efficacy, safety, and use in clinical and preclinical applications." *Alternative Therapy and Health Medicine.* 2001, May–Jun: 7(3)93–100.

Milewicz, A., Gejdel, E. and H. Sworen. "*Vitex agnus castus* extract in the treatment of luteal phase defects due to latent hyperprolactinemia. Results of a randomized placebo-controlled double-blind study." *Arzneimittelforschung.* 1993 Jul: 43(7)752–756.

Mizunuma, H., Kanazawa, K., Ogura, S., et al. "Anticarcinogenic effects of isoflavones may be mediated by genistein in mouse mammary tumor virus-induced breast cancer." *Oncology.* 2002: 62(1)78–84.

Mohr, P.E., Wang, D.Y., Gregory, W.M., et al. "Serum progesterone and prognosis in operable breast cancer." *British Journal of Cancer.* 1996: (73)1552–1555.

Murray, Michael, N.D. *Encyclopedia of Natural Medicine.* 2nd ed. (Prima Publishing, 1997).

"'Natural' progesterone creams for postmenopausal women." *Drug Therapy Bulletin.* 2001, Feb: 39(2)10–11.

Nestel, P. "Isoflavones from red clover improve systemic arterial compliance but not plasma lipids in menopausal women." *Journal of Clinical Endocrinology Metabolism.* 1999, Mar: 84(3)895–898

North American Menopause Society. "The role of isoflavones in menopausal health: consensus opinion of the North American Menopause Society." *Menopause.* 2000, Jul–Aug: 7(4)215–229.

Petitti, D.B. "Hormone replacement therapy for prevention: more evidence, more pessimism." *JAMA* 2002 Jun-July: 49(6):641-2.

Pick, M. "Herbal treatments for menopause. Black cohosh, soy and micronized progesterone." *Advanced Nurse Practitioner.* 2000 May: 8(5)29–30.

Ratna, W.N. "Inhibition of estrogenic stimulation of gene expression by genistein." *Life Science.* 2002, Jul 12: 71(8)865–877.

Ribom, E., Piehl-Aulin, K., Ljunghall, S., Ljunggren, O. and T. Naessen. "Six months of hormone replacement therapy does not influence muscle strength in postmenopausal women." *Maturitas.* 2002, Jul 25: 42(3)225.

Riis, B.J., Thomsen, K., Strom, V. and C. Christiansen. "The effect of percutaneous estradiol and natural progesterone on postmenopausal bone loss." *American Journal of Obstetrics and Gynecology.* 1987: (156)61–65.

Rosano, G.M., Webb, C.M., Chierchia, S., et al. "Natural progesterone, but not medroxyprogesterone acetate, enhances the beneficial effect of estrogen on exercise-induced myocardial ischemia in postmenopausal women." *J Am Coll Cardiol.* 2000, Dec: 36(7)2154–2159.

Schellenberg, R. "Treatment for the premenstrual syndrome with agnus castus fruit extract: prospective, randomised, placebo controlled study." *British Medical Journal.* 2001, Jan 20: 322(7279)134–137.

Shao, Z., Wu, J. and Z. Shen. "Genistein exerts multiple suppressive effects on human breast carcinoma cells." *Zhonghua Zhong Liu Za Zhi.* 2000 Sep: 22(5)362–365.

Shao, Z. and Z. Shen. "Mechanism of growth inhibition by genistein of human breast carcinoma." *Zhonghua Zhong Liu Za Zhi.* 1999 Sep: 21(5)325–328.

Solomon, Neil, M.D., et al. *Soy Smart Health.* (Woodland, 2000).

Somjen, D., Amir-Zaltsman, Y., Gayer, B. et al. "6-Carboxymethyl genistein: a novel selective oestrogen receptor modulator (SERM) with unique, differential effects on the vasculature, bone and uterus." *Journal of Endocrinology.* 2002, Jun: 173(3)415–427.

Steinberg, S. et al. "A placebo-controlled clinical trial of L-tryptophan in premenstrual dysphoria." *Biological Psychiatry.* 1999, Feb 1: 45(3)313–20.

Stephens, C. "The relationship between hormone replacement therapy use and psychological symptoms: no effects found in a New Zealand sample." *Health Care Women International.* 2002, Jun: 23(4)408–414.

Stevinson, C. and E. Ernst. "A pilot study of Hypericum perforatum for the treatment of premenstrual syndrome." *British Journal of Obstetrics and Gynecology.* 2000, Jul: 107(7)870–876.

Tripathi, B.K., Gupta, B. and A.K. Agarwal. "Adverse effects of hormone replacement therapy."

Tsunoda, N., Pomeroy, S. and P. Nestel. "Absorption in humans of isoflavones from soy and red clover is similar." *Journal of Nutrition.* 2002, Aug: 132(8)2199–2201.

Van de Weijer, P. and R. Barentsen. "Isoflavones from red clover (Promensil(R)) significantly reduce menopausal hot flush symptoms compared with placebo." *Maturitas.* 2002, Jul 25: 42(3)187.

Vastag, B. "Hormone replacement therapy falls out of favor with expert committee." *Journal of the American Medical Association.* 2002, Apr 17: 287(15)1923–1924.

Vincent, A. and L.A. Fitzpatrick. "Soy isoflavones: are they useful in menopause?" *Mayo Clinic Procedures.* 2000, Nov: 75(11)1174–1184.

Yan, C. and R. Han. "Protein tyrosine kinase inhibitor genistein suppresses in vitro invasion of HT1080 human fibrosarcoma cells." *Zhonghua Zhong Liu Za Zhi.* 1999, May: 21(3)171–174.

For more information on the National Institutes of Health (NIH)'s Women's Health Initiative (WHI) contact:

Women's Health Initiative Program Office
1 Rockledge Centre
Suite 300, MS 7966
6705 Rockledge Drive
Bethesda, Maryland 20892-7966
Phone: (301) 402-2900
Fax: (301) 480-5158
On the web: www.nhlbi.nih.gov/whi/

About the Author

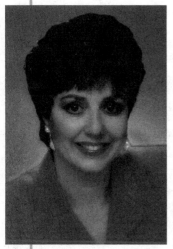

RITA ELKINS, M.H., has worked as an author and research specialist in the health field for the last ten years, and possesses a strong background in both conventional and alternative health therapies. She is the author of numerous books, including *Solving the Depression Puzzle,* which provides an in-depth look at overcoming the complex problem of depression, *The Pocket Herbal Reference, The Complete Fiber Fact Book,* and *The Herbal Emergency Guide.* Rita has also authored dozens of booklets exploring the documented value of natural supplements like SAMe, noni, blue-green algae, chitosan, stevia and many more. She received an honorary Master Herbalist Degree from the College of Holistic Health and Healing in 1994.

Rita is frequently consulted for the formulation of herbal blends and is a frequent host on radio talk shows exploring natural health topics. She is also a regular contributor to *Let's Live* and *Great Life* magazines. She lectures nationwide on the science behind natural compounds and collaborates with medical doctors on various projects. Rita's publications and lectures have been used by companies like Nature's Sunshine, 4-Life Research, Enrich, and NuSkin to support the credibility of natural and integrative health therapies. She recently co-authored *Soy Smart Health* with *New York Times'* best-selling author Neil Solomon, M.D., and *A Maverick of Medicine Speaks to Women,* with Duane Townsend, M.D.

Rita resides in Utah, is married, and has two daughters and two granddaughters.

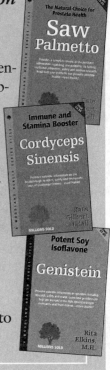

Fight osteoporosis and heart disease with

Natural Alternatives to HRT

As the risks of conventional synthetic HRT become more apparent, more and more women are turning to natural alternatives for relief of menopausal complaints and postmenopausal disease such as osteoporosis and heart disease. In fact, there are a number of proven natural menopausal remedies including the soy isoflavone, genistein, natural progesterone cream and a number of beneficial herbal medicines. Dietary changes and certain types of exercise also provide a number of health benefits for menopausal women without the use of dangerous drugs. Read inside to find out how you can take advantage of safe and effective natural alternatives to HRT.

OTHER BOOKLETS IN THE WOODLAND HEALTH SERIES

- Natural Cold/Flu Defense • Kava Kava
- Chinese Red Yeast Rice • CLA • Olive Leaf
- Suppl. for Fibromyalgia • SAM-e • 5-HTP
- Conquering Caffeine Dependence • DHA

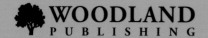

WOODLAND
PUBLISHING

50495

9 781580 543699

ISBN 1-58054-369-3